New Every Morning

by Earline Kline

A Devotional for caregivers

and their patients.

New Every Morning

By

Earline Kline

A Devotional for Caregivers

And their Patients

ISBN   978-0-9960146-9-4

Interior Design: Endurance Press
Cover Design: Teal Rose Design Studio's

Dedicated to John and Vivian Wilcox.

Foreword

Dan and I were in prison ministry for twenty years. It was always our dream that one day, when Dan retired, he could become a prison chaplain.

When a dear friend moved from the maximum-security prison to the medium- security prison, Dan was given the chaplain's position at the maximum prison. Our hearts were filled with so much joy as God had given us the desire of our hearts. Then, thirteen months later, the Idaho Chaplain's Corp came to our home and removed Dan from his position. We were crushed.

It seemed Dan had developed a habit of being forgetful, as well as several other strange behaviors. Before I finally fell asleep that night, I said to the Lord: "I have to have a word from You." The first words in my mind as I awoke the next morning were: "The clouds you so much dread, will break with blessing on your head." And, after caring for my mother, I dreaded Alzheimer's. God was promising Dan's Alzheimer's would be a blessing in our lives. I clung to that promise for the next six and a half years, until Dan went home to Glory.

Earline

God Never Wastes Anything

$$\sim\!\!\times\!\!\sim$$

"And we know that in all things God works for the good of those who love Him, who have been called according to His purpose." Romans 8:28

All of us are going to face difficult times in our lives. When this verse was written, the Jews were facing extremely difficult persecution. Paul wrote to encourage them in their trials. He assured them they were safe in God's love, and that nothing that happened to them could ever separate them from that love. "*Neither life nor death, nor things present, or things to come.*" That about covers all the bases. Paul's words promised the Jews that: "*the sufferings of this present time are not worth comparing to the glory that is to come.*" He holds out great hope for them, and for us who are suffering today.

8

There is nothing in your life that happens to you that God cannot turn for your good. Even the sinful, hurtful acts of others against you. Remember Joseph, whose brothers sold him into slavery? Even there, God blessed him. Joseph could later say: *"You meant it for evil, but God meant it for good; for the saving of many people alive."* Their very sin would later save their lives, and the lives of many others. Egyptians included.

God is so amazing! Stand back and watch Him take your present pain, trials, and difficulties, and build your character and make you more like Jesus. That's God's ultimate goal in your life.

Action Step: Trust God, even when it hurts. Even when the way is dark. He is at work accomplishing His purposes in your life.

Don't Sweat the Big Stuff

"Then Moses stretched out his hand over the sea, and all that night the Lord drove the sea back with a strong east wind, and turned it into dry land. The waters were divided and the Israelites went through the sea on dry ground..."
Exodus 14:21-22a

Israel had just left Egypt after four hundred years of slavery, and they were camped by the Red Sea. Pharaoh had decided to pursue them and his army was camped behind them. They couldn't go forward, they couldn't go backward. They were facing the impossible. God's instructions were to sit still and watch Him work. So, Moses stretched out his rod over the sea, and God parted the waters and made a path through the sea. The Israelites crossed on dry ground, safely, to the other side.

I call those huge impossible situations the Red Sea places of my life, and God has seen me through many of them.

I've found the greater the problem, the greater the miracle. It is best if I just sit still and let Him work in His way and His time. It is easy to leave the big problems in His hands because I know I can't solve them.

Action Step: Sit still and trust God to see you through the impossible situations of your life.

Don't Sweat the Small Stuff

❦✕❧

"Are not two sparrows sold for a penny? Yet not one of them will fall to the ground apart from the will of your Father. And even the very hairs of your head are all numbered." Matthew 10: 29-30

God cares about the big events of my life and takes care of the smallest details. I'm always tempted to take small matters into my own hands. I think, "I can handle this," rather than committing it to God.

I love to see Him work in the small things. I feel His love more when He does small, unexpected acts.

Pick your battles with your Alzheimer's patient. Ask yourself, "Does it really matter? Can I just back off and let it slide? Do I really need to get so upset when he or she does something out of the ordinary?"

I learned to simplify life for Dan, as much as possible, as he struggled through his Alzheimer's: putting out only one piece of silverware that he needed for his meal, buying boneless chicken, and seedless watermelon.

I kept to a set routine; kept him in what was familiar to him. No sudden changes. Because of that, we were actually able to be in the prison, doing our prayer group, six weeks before Dan died.

Action Step: Commit the small things to God. Look for ways to simplify life for your loved one.

Lean Hard on God

"Trust in the Lord with all your heart, and lean not on your own understanding; in all your ways acknowledge Him, and He will make your paths straight." Proverbs 3:5,6

When my sister asked me to care for my mother who had Alzheimer's, I wasn't sure I could do it. I had never cared for an elderly person, let alone someone who had memory loss.

But I said yes, and found I could do what I thought I couldn't do. God was faithful to help me day by day.

Sometimes I would wake up in the night, and sense a presence in my room. Mom would be standing quietly beside my bed. I would get up and gently put her back in her bed. She would have crying jags, and weep and weep, unable to tell me what was the matter. I would sit by her side with my arm around her until the weeping subsided.

I am a goal setter and a list maker. It is hard for me to totally lean on God, but it is necessary.

My confidence grew after caring for my mom, and my husband's Alzheimer's diagnosis brought a sense of knowing that I could care for him also.

Action Step: Don't lean on your own understanding. Choose to lean hard on God and trust Him in the hard places of life.

Live One Day at a Time

"Therefore, do not worry about tomorrow, for tomorrow will worry about itself. Each day has enough trouble of its own."
Matthew 6:25-34

As I learned to live with a husband with Alzheimer's, I learned to live in day tight compartments. I would tell myself: "I can live with how Dan is today." I dared not think about what the next tomorrow might bring. My mind could imagine all kinds of things, none of them good. I had watched my mom deteriorate with Alzheimer's and I knew the same thing would happen to Dan.

Dan and I continued our prison prayer group until just six weeks before he died. I drove us out to the prison, signed us in and out and did all the talking, as Dan could no longer do those things. The men loved him so much; his presence and smile enough for them.

16

I visualized being confined to my home caring for Dan. That never happened. I visualized closing my daycare. I never had to close the doors, and Dan and little Kaden continued to love each other immensely. Most of the bad things I visualized never happened.

Action Step: Live in day tight compartments. Don't borrow tomorrow's worry or pain. Take one day at a time.

Meet with God Daily

*"O God, thou art my God; early will I seek thee: my soul
thirsteth for thee, my flesh longeth for thee; in a dry and thirsty
land, where no water is." Psalm 63:1*

As a caregiver, it is so important to begin your day with God. Draw on His grace and strength. Out of His abundant supply He has promised enough for whatever your day will bring. Set your heart and mind on Him. Be quiet before Him and listen for His gentle whisper.

Dan had a couple knee replacement surgeries during the Alzheimer's years. Immediately after the first surgery, we lost Dan completely mentally. He could not communicate with us at all. I was called to the hospital and had to stay right beside him, holding his hand to keep him calm and in bed. In the early morning hours, I wept and prayed, begging God to give him back to me as he was before the surgery.

That second afternoon, a patient sitter arrived to sit with Dan. He informed me that he was a retired Nazarene pastor. We shared across Dan's bedside all afternoon. Just before I left for the evening, I asked him to pray with us. I felt free to leave, as I knew Dan would be in good hands. And, God did give Dan back to me as he had been before his surgery.

Action Step: Keep your heart in tune with God by meeting with Him everyday. Cling to His presence.

Find Those Quiet Resting Places

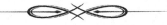

"He makes me lie down in green pastures, He leads me beside quiet waters, He restores my soul. He guides me in paths of righteousness for His name's sake." Psalm 23:2-3

Learn what restores your soul. A nap, losing yourself in a good book or movie, lunch with a friend, a telephone conversation with someone you love, praying with your prayer partner.

I have a dear friend who prays with me over the phone. I love to hear her pray for me. It lifts and encourages me. I now have a special place I love to go. It is quiet and serene. I sit on a stone bench near a tumbling stream and just talk to God, and let all my cares go. Peace, like a river, floods my soul. I never dreamed when we buried Dan on that little hillside, that it would become such a special place for me.

When you really need to get away for a few hours, there are volunteer organizations out there that will send someone to your home to be with your loved one. Find them; use them, so you can have some soul restoration time.

Taking care of yourself is very important if you are going to be the caregiver your loved one needs.

Action Step: Take care of yourself. Find what restores your soul and make time for it in your life.

When Depressed, Read Psalms

"The Lord is faithful to all His promises, and loving toward all He has made. The Lord upholds all those who fall, and lifts up all who are bowed down." Psalm 145: 13b-14

There are times when life just plain gets you down. David knew what that was like, and he penned many of the Psalms. He poured out his heart in poetry. Often, he began with complaining and anger, and ended with praise.

Every cry of your heart can be found in the Psalms. When depressed, read until you find the words to express your feelings. Read and pray through the Psalms until you are thanking and praising God.

I have so much arthritis and deal with so much pain in my joints; so I, too, cry out: *"O Lord, heal me, for my bones are in agony." (Psalm 6:2b)*

When I was depressed, I memorized Psalm 42, 43, and 51. I lived in those three Psalms for a year, confident I would praise God again and that He would restore my joy. And He did.

When Dan was in the hospital near the end of his life, I would read the Psalms to him. I would start with Psalms 23 and go on from there, everyday.

Action Step: Spend some time every day in the Psalms. Stay there until God lifts you up and you can thank and praise Him.

Give Thanks in All Things

———⟨✕⟩———

"Be joyful always, pray continually, give thanks in all cir-
cumstances, for this is God's will for you in Christ Jesus."
1 Thessalonians 5:16-18

Give thanks for Dan's Alzheimer's? I cried out to God:
"Lord, I can't do that. Not in myself. It's going to take a
Spirit stronger than me." The reply always came: "I have
given you my Holy Spirit, child. He will enable you to give
thanks."

When you start giving thanks, sometimes things change
immediately, and sometimes, you are simply given the
strength to go on.

I remember the days I was in so much physical pain. I
would fall on my knees and beg God for relief and heal-
ing. Though nothing changed, I would find strength to

24

go on. I really don't know how I got through those days, with four daycare children. The pain was in my head often times, and head pain makes it very hard to function. Eventually, the head pain, which often caused pain in my ear and jaw, was relieved by the dentist.

We have a choice. We can go through life complaining, or we can go through life giving thanks for everything. If you can't give God thanks for what is happening, thank Him for who He is and what He does.

Action Step: Make it a habit of life to give God thanks, no matter what is happening. He is still the blessed controller of all things.

Stay Focused on Jesus

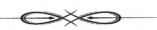

"...let us run with perseverance the race marked out for us. Let us fix our eyes on Jesus, the author and perfector of our faith, who, for the joy set before Him, endured the cross, scorning its shame, and sat down at the right hand of the throne of God."
Hebrews 12:1b-2

If you have cared for or watched someone deteriorate from Alzheimer's, as I watched my mother, then you know some of the things ahead of you. If I thought about what would happen to Dan and counted the losses, it would have totally overwhelmed me. When I considered that all the decisions would fall on me, it seemed like a heavy burden. Dan had always done all the household repairs and taken care of the car. How would I know when the car needed repairs? Would it tell me?

How would I run this race through Alzheimer's? By keeping my eyes fixed on Jesus, not my circumstances, not

26

on what could happen; but by praying to God through it all.

Jesus endured the cross by focusing on what the cross would accomplish, the joy of bringing many sons into glory. We can do the same, knowing we are becoming more Christ-like by caring for our weak loved one.

Action Step: Keep your eyes fixed on Jesus, not the circumstances in which you find yourself.

Learn to Laugh

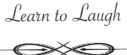

"A cheerful heart is good medicine, but a crushed spirit dries up the bones." Proverbs 17:22

Dan and I would share cooking breakfast together. On pancake day, I would cook my pancake and put my egg on to cook in the little skillet, and Dan's pancake in the large skillet. Dan would turn my egg and his pancake. This particular morning, when it came time to turn my egg, Dan took the skillet and flipped my egg over onto the burner. I jumped up and began to clean the burner. Then when it came time to turn his pancake, he took the skillet and again, flipped the food onto the burner. I cried out: "Are you using your brain?!" Immediately I was sorry, and proceeded to clean up the second burner. Needless to say, Dan had something else for breakfast, and that ended his helping me in the kitchen.

When I got to support group and told the story of our Alzheimer's breakfast, we laughed until tears flowed. It may not have been funny at the time, but the more I told the story, the funnier it got.

I kept a journal, and wrote everything down in those Alzheimer's years, so I wouldn't forget it. Sometimes those memories and moments became cause for laughter.

Action Step: Don't let yourself get too upset about the strange things that your loved one does. Choose to laugh instead.

Listen to Wise Counsel

"For by wise counsel thou shalt make thy war: and in multitude of counselors there is safety." Proverbs 24:6

I was determined not to put Dan in a nursing home. He was sent to one for rehab after his second knee replacement surgery, and I could hardly stand seeing him there.

We celebrated our fiftieth wedding anniversary in July, and all the children were home. We had a glorious weekend together. Dan really began to go downhill after that. He was getting me up four and five times a night, and there would be puddles of urine on the bathroom floor. I now had to help him dress and shower.

Near Thanksgiving, Dan developed a urinary tract infection and we had to take him to the emergency room. He was in the hospital for five days. When it came time to move him, he wasn't mobile. I knew I couldn't handle him at home. My son told me: "Mom, it's time."

I ended up putting him back I the same nursing home where he had completed his rehab. That was the hardest thing I had ever done. I cried all the way home. Things don't turn out as hoped and planned, and sometimes, big decisions make themselves.

Action Step: Seek God's face and counsel and listen to those around you. What looks so terrible may prove to be a great blessing.

Do the Hard Thing: A Care Facility

"...I have learned the secret of being content in any and every circumstance, whether well-fed or hungry, whether living in plenty or in want. I can do everything through Him who gives me strength." Philippians 4:12b-13

God gives us strength to do the hard things in life. Placing Dan in a care facility was probably the most difficult thing I had to do, but I realized I couldn't care for him at home any longer. He never walked again, or fed himself again. I was still doing daycare, but only had two children. I had a son and a grandson living with me, and I would prepare their meals in the evenings, and then drive to the nursing home to feed Dan.

Dan was surrounded by Christian nurses and aides. Even the woman in the office was a believer. His evening nurse was a very fine and caring young man. I left Dan with tears the day I took him to the nursing home, telling him: "Honey, I can't care for you anymore."

Dan knew us until the very last days. On Monday, when I bent over to kiss him, he pursed his lips for my kiss. He knew I was there. On Thursday, he graduated to Glory, and our long battle with Alzheimer's was over. Dan's race, and mine with him, was complete.

Action Step: Things probably won't go as you desire or expect. Be open to all God has for you in these days of caregiving.

Ask For Wisdom

*"If any of you lacks wisdom, let him ask God, who gives gener-
ously to all, without finding fault, and it will be given to him."*
James 1:5

Do you feel overwhelmed with the decisions you have to
make? Decisions you and your mate always made together? Now this whole load falls on you, and it seems to be
way too much.

I remember the day the car wouldn't start. No Dan
to help me, so I called Les Schwab and they came and
jump- started my car. I then drove to their store and had
a new battery installed. I was amazed that I had handled
a problem like that by myself. I gained a lot of confidence,
and I realized, yes, the car would tell me if something was
wrong.

I remember sharing a piece of writing with Dan, needing his input, though I realized he would be of little help. Old habits die hard.

I actually purchased a car all on my own, the last week of Dan's life. I sought counsel from everyone, and prayed a lot. God guided me each step of the way and gave me the desire of my heart. When the salesman drove up that light blue Toyota Camry, I knew it was my car. There was no doubt in my mind. Even my sons said: "You did good, Mom."

Action Step: When you need help with decisions, seek the wisdom of God. He is more than willing to give it to you.

Rely on the Holy Spirit Within

"But the fruit of the spirit is love, joy, peace, patience, kindness, goodness, faithfulness, gentleness, and self-control. Against such things there is no law." Galatians 5:22

When Dan was diagnosed with Alzheimer's, he told everybody around him. I was deep in denial for months. It was a difficult thing to face after caring for my mother and watching what the Alzheimer's did to her.

When I cared for my mom the first time, I wasn't sure I could do it. But, I discovered I could do what I thought was too hard. I had prayed that Alzheimer's wouldn't happen to us, but it did. I had prayed I would never have arthritis as I can't take the drugs, but I'm full of arthritic pain.

With Dan's diagnosis, I knew God had some special

work to do in the garden of my life. I felt He was going to especially work on making me a more gentle person.

The fruit of the spirit is in you at all times. You need to draw upon His love, patience, kindness, and gentleness, as you care for your loved one. Start everyday yielding to the Holy Spirit asking Him to fill you and control you, to bring forth His fruit in your life.

Action Step: Live a spirit-filled, spirit controlled life, and the fruit of your garden will be beautiful.

Build a Network of Support

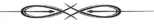

"As Jesus walked beside the Sea of Galilee, He saw Simon and his brother Andrew casting a net into the lake, for they were fishermen. 'Come, follow me,' Jesus said. 'and I will make you fishers of men.' At once, they left their nets and followed Him."
Mark 1:16-18

If ever you needed someone to walk beside you, it is when your loved one has Alzheimer's. Dan and I joined an Alzheimer's support group and met with them the last two years of his life. At our meetings we divided into patients and caregivers. Dan would come home so encouraged. I found others dealing with different things and I could really let my hair down. I made decisions in that group that would carry me through Dan's last days. One decision: we would take away the drugs once he was in a nursing home and let the Alzheimer's take its course. Actually our doctor did that.

I developed a network to take care of the house: plumber, electrician, carpenter, air conditioning, and furnace man. We have Handyman Connection here and I have used them also.

I had a dear friend I could sit down and have a cup of tea with and share my week, and a friend to pray with me over the phone.

Action Step: Build a support group around you to walk with you through the Alzheimer's days.

Memorial Stones: Keep a Journal

"...go over before the ark of the Lord your God into the middle of the Jordan. Each of you is to take up a stone on his shoulder, according to the number of tribes of the Israelites, to serve as a sign among you." Joshua 4:5-6a

My son said early to write down everything in a journal. If I hadn't written the Alzheimer's breakfast story, I couldn't have remembered it correctly. There were many other instances as Alzheimer's patients do many strange things. For example, not putting the frozen blueberries in the freezer but putting them on the garage floor. Or, the toothpaste ending up in the pantry with the canned goods, instead of in the bathroom. I also watched Dan attempt to wash his hands in the toilet, fussing because he couldn't find the soap.

When Dan was still cooking, one morning, instead of

cutting up ham to put in our waffles, he cut up smoked turkey lunch- meat. The waffles just didn't taste the same.

You must have an ID to get into the prison. Somehow Dan misplaced his but they let him in anyway. I finally found it in his coat pocket. One more loss for him as I now had to carry it for him.

Action Step: Write everything down in a journal. You'll be glad you did. It may get funnier with the telling.

Remember God's Past Faithfulness

───────❈───────

"I will remember the deeds of the Lord; Yes, I will remember your miracles of long ago. I will meditate on all your works and consider all your mighty deeds." Psalms 77:11-12

This is so important. Remembering how God has worked in the past will give you the courage for all your tomorrows.

We've had a lot of financial difficulties but when I remember past miracles of provision by a faithful God, I know I can trust Him for the next hard place.

People say: "I don't know how you went through caring for your husband." One person told me: "Alzheimer's is a terrible disease." I just went through it one day at a time and trusted God for the grace to get through that day. The little children in the daycare helped a lot. They were our joy and Dan never got mean with them as my mother did. I remember having to tell my sister I couldn't care for our mother anymore after that.

Kaden was a toddler, and a real sweetheart, in the group of children at my daycare. He loved Dan and would crawl up in his lap. Dan loved him.

Remember, God has never failed you in the past, and He will not fail you whatever the future may bring.

Action Step: When you are tempted to doubt God's care for today and tomorrow, remember His past faithfulness. He cannot fail you.

No More Than You Can Bear

"No temptation has seized you except what is common to man. And God is faithful; He will not let you be tempted beyond what you can bear. But when you are tempted, He will also provide a way out so that you can stand up under it."
1 Corinthians 10:13

No matter what you go through, someone has been there before you. You are not alone. It may feel like it, because Alzheimer's tends to isolate you. You need to keep your loved one in a set routine and in places familiar to them. That is why I wanted to keep Dan in our home. Yet, I changed churches the last year of his life and moved him from a small church to a large one, and he did just fine. We joined a small group Bible study, and they welcomed us with open arms.

You may think this is more than you can handle, yet God promises it won't be. He will provide a way through, even if it is just a change of attitude. If you need a break, have someone come in for an afternoon and go out to lunch with a friend.

The changes were so gradual with Dan, I hardly noticed them. As he needed more and more help, I just stepped up and did what was required.

Action Step: Realize God is with you all the way with special grace for each hour, each day. It won't be more than you can bear.

Rejoice in the Trial

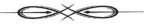

"Consider it pure joy, my brothers, whenever you face trials of many kinds, because you know that the testing of your faith produces perseverance. Perseverance must finish its work so that you may be complete, not lacking anything." James 1:2-4

Consider my current trial pure joy? James, what are you saying? How can I count this pain pure joy? I'd much rather complain. I know it is going to take a power greater than myself to rejoice in this pain. I will have to depend on the Holy Spirit.

When I know God is cutting and polishing me through my trials so that I might better reflect Jesus, that is pure joy.

Let patience have her perfect work. I need to submit to God's work in my life and let Him bring me to maturity. The joy is becoming more like Jesus through the very trials I want to escape.

46

God's purpose in our lives is not to make us comfortable but to build our character, and He does that through the trials we face.

Don't give up if you fail the test. God will send another and another until you finally pass.

Action Step: Determine to rejoice in your trials, and let patience have her perfect work in you. Only then will you become more like Christ.

He Knows All About Me

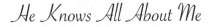

"O Lord, you have searched me and you know me. You know when I sit and when I rise; you perceive my thoughts from afar." Psalm 139:1-2

Rest in this: God knows you through and through. He knows when you reach the end of your strength and need a break. He knows your thoughts before you think them; every word in your mouth before you speak it. He knows how demanding caregiving is.

He knows how tiring it was to care for children all day, feed my family, then rush to the nursing home to feed Dan, and stay until they put him to bed. He knew I could not handle a long nursing home stay. So after five short weeks, He took Dan home.

God balances the blessings and the trials in our lives. He

knows our strengths and our weaknesses. He sings over us songs of deliverance, rejoices when we trust Him for strength, surrounds us with His love, and pours out His mercies on us.

The words of an old song say: "When we have exhausted our store of endurance, when our strength has failed ere the day is half done, when we reach the end of our hoarded resources, our Father's full giving is only begun."

Action Step: God knows what you are going through right now and He gives more grace when the burdens grow greater.

Worship

"At this, Job got up and tore his robe and shaved his head. Then he fell to the ground in worship and said: 'Naked I came from my Mother's womb, and naked I will depart. The Lord gave and the Lord has taken away; may the name of the Lord be praised.'" Job 1:20-21

Tragedy had fallen on Job; perhaps more than any man should have to bear. All six of his children were killed, and all his flocks and herds were destroyed. What was Job's reaction? He did not give up his faith, but fell on his face and worshipped God.

When my dad died of a heart attack, my brother, even in his grief, began to pour out his heart in worship in the early morning hours when he could not sleep.

God has not changed, no matter what befalls us. We can still praise and thank Him for who He is and what He does. He is still the blessed controller of all things. He is still full of loving-kindness, full of mercy, and faithful to keep His promises. He is still the God of the impossible; able to do exceedingly abundantly above all we can ask or imagine.

Action Step: You have been slammed with the totally unexpected. Like Job, fall on your knees in worship.

When You Pass Through the Waters

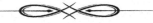

"When you pass through the waters, I will be with you. And when you pass through the rivers, they will not sweep over you. When you walk through the fire, you will not be burned; the flames will not set you ablaze." Isaiah 43:2

There have been times in my life I have cried out like David: "All your waves and billows have gone over me." I was sure I could not handle what was coming at me, and was convinced I would drown. At those times, I clung to this promise in Isaiah. I realized I was not alone. God was with me. He is always a present tense God. The Great I AM.

Here, God is promising to walk through the trial with you. He promises that it will not overwhelm you. And, He promises to bring you safely to the other side.

We are either entering a trial, in the midst of one, or coming out of one. It is in the trials of life that God becomes so real to us that we experience His mercies the most. We can sense His love for us, and experience His miracles. God meets us at the desperation points of life. He delights in meeting the needs of His children, and hearing their thankful praises.

Action Step: Get alone, get a promise, get quiet and listen for the gentle whisper of God. He's saying: "I AM with you."

Jesus Comes to us in The Storm

"But when they saw Him walking on the lake, they thought He was a ghost. They cried out, because they all saw Him and were terrified. Immediately He spoke to them and said, 'Take courage! It is I! Don't be afraid.'" Mark 6:49-50

Jesus comes to us in the storms of life, walking on the very waves that threaten us. The Gospel of Mark tells us: *"Jesus saw them toiling in the rowing."* That tells us Jesus sees in the dark. He sees us in our struggles when all is dark and we can't see any way out. He comes and stills the storm in our hearts, speaking peace to our troubled thoughts.

There is no storm He cannot still, no turmoil of the soul He can't calm with a word from Him. He is the author of peace.

In Psalm 107, we find God brings the storm into our lives. When we cry out to Him in our storm, He comes to us and delivers us. Then we give thanks for His unfailing love and wonderful deeds.

Storms are going to come; often suddenly and unexpectedly. They catch us off guard, but God is never surprised. They are all a part of His plan for us. Reach out your hand and grasp His. He is there in the darkness with you.

Action Step: When you can't see His face, trust His heart. He loves you too much to let you drown.

Anger

"In your anger do not sin. When you are on your beds, search your hearts and be silent. Offer right sacrifices and trust in the Lord." Psalm 4:4-5

Anger can be a very real part of caregiving. My sister cared for our mom for eleven years. I helped her as I could until it became impossible due to the demands of my daycare. Now her husband has Alzheimer's also, and she is suffering from anger at having to go through the entire process again.

You may become angry at siblings who won't, or can't help care for an aging parent, thus causing the load to fall on you. You may be angry when you see what the disease is doing to your loved one. Alzheimer's is a disease of losses, and you grieve each one.

Dan lost his ability to communicate verbally early in his diagnosis. He also lost much of his common sense. We struggled with communication all the time. Much of the time I could figure out what he was trying to say, and other times we both just gave up in frustration. I learned to let things go when they weren't worth fighting over. Those fights left us both upset, and that outcome wasn't worth it.

So, give up anger and accept God's grace for the moment.

Action Step: Choose your battles. Some things are not worth fighting over. Ask yourself: "Does it really matter?"

Pour Out Your Heart

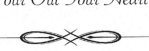

"Trust in Him at all times, O people; Pour out your heart before Him. For God is our refuge." Psalm 62:8

There are times in your caregiving when your heart just becomes so full of frustration, grief, and anger that you need to pour it out before God. God is not surprised at your feelings and you need the release.

You may go to the Psalms again and find expression for what you are feeling. Pray the words back to God and stay there until you can praise Him again.

When I knew I was losing Dan, I couldn't sleep in the early morning hours. I just wept and prayed, pouring my heart out before God, feeling my loss. It wasn't until I stopped focusing on my loss and started focusing on God that my heart had rest.

God lead me to Psalm 63 on Christmas morning. There I found comfort. Four days later Dan would graduate to glory.

God welcomes the pouring out of our hearts before Him, and He, in turn, fills us up with His comfort. Listen for His whisper in the darkness: *I am here, child.*

Action Step: When my heart is overwhelmed, lead me to the Rock that is higher than I. I will pour out my heart before You.

Cling to the Promises

"Remember your word to your servant, for you have given me hope. My comfort in my suffering is this: Your promise renews my life." Psalm 119:49-50

Remember the word God gave me when I suspected Dan had Alzheimer's? "The clouds you so much dread, are great with mercy, and will break with blessing over your head." They are the words of an old hymn. God has often spoken to me through the words of songs.

When we faced the move from California to Idaho, the Lord told us: "Be not dismayed what'er betide, God will take care of you." My heart quieted as I trusted in His promise.

Be quiet before Him and listen for His voice. He has a special promise for you today. He cannot lie and He is the great promise keeper.

When I knew I was going to Israel alone as a volunteer, I clung to a select few promises. Joshua 1:9: that God would be with me, and Isaiah 41:10: that God would give me strength to work in the soup kitchen. To quiet my fears and doubts, I reviewed these verses daily. God was faithful even though I missed my connection at the airport on my arrival.

Action Step: Get ready to listen. God has a promise to fit your situation today. Cling to it with all your might.

Cast All Your Cares on Him

*"Humble yourselves, therefore, under God's mighty hand, that
He may lift you up in due time. Cast all your anxiety upon
Him because He cares for you." 1 Peter 5:6-7*

I find it difficult at times, to cast all my cares on Jesus,
even though I know I must. Especially when it concerns
my children and their decision -making. I know it weighs
me down and I need to cast it on Jesus, otherwise I will
never know peace.

I need to obey Philipians 4:6:

*"Do not be anxious about anything, but in everything, by
prayer and petition, and with thanksgiving, present your
requests to God. And the peace of God will guard your heart
and mind in Christ Jesus."*

I need to be convinced of God's care for me and
my children. I need to remember how God cared for me

in Israel; how I was shown kindness from perfect strangers, how I was rescued by taxi drivers when I was stranded; for someone who spoke English to me when I was in need of assistance.

So remember, God's past miracles of care in the big things and in the smallest details.

Action Step: Literally throw the weight of all your cares on Jesus. He is able to carry them much better than you.

Sing in the Shadow of His Wings

❈

"On my bed I remember you; I think of you through the watch of night. Because you are my help, I sing in the shadow of your wings." Psalm 63:6-7

Shortly before Dan died, God gave me Psalm 63, and I was determined to sing in the shadow of His wings.

Today I asked God for a song to sing its way through my mind all day long. He gave me: "His name is a mighty tower."

In Colossians 3, Paul speaks of being filled with God's word, and singing it back to Him in psalms, hymns, and spiritual songs. Most worship choruses we sing today are singing God's word back to Him. What a great way to worship and be reminded of His truths.

Moses taught the children of Israel a song so they would

remember God's truth. I believe we will actually sing the song of Moses in heaven.

Paul and Silas sang hymns and prayed at midnight with their feet in stocks in the inner prison, and with their backs bloodied and bruised. God shook that prison and freed them, and the even the jailor and his family.

Ask God for a song in the night. It may deliver you from your anxiety and fears.

Action Step: Put on a praise cd and sing along with it. Your spirit will be lifted into heartfelt thanksgiving.

He Remembers That I am Dust

"As a father has compassion on his children, so the Lord has compassion on those who fear Him. For He knows how we are formed, He remembers that we are dust." Psalm 103:13-14

I am so thankful God remembers how human and weak I am. He doesn't expect the world of me, just simple obedience. He knows I'll make mistakes and He takes the messes I make and brings good out of them.

I really angered a taxi driver in Israel after not waiting for him. Even though I paid for a trip I didn't take, I don't think he will ever forgive me. I just had to give my mistake to God and trust Him to bring good out of it.

I don't have a lot of strength, so I knew I would have to trust God to be able to work in the soup kitchen in Israel. I reminded God that He was sending a weak vessel to serve there, but I also knew that God chooses to work through our weaknesses. So I obeyed and went, and God was faithful to help me. One day a young couple from Holland urged me to go home and rest.

God doesn't expect perfection, only obedience. He remembers that we are dust.

Action Step: We need to remember we are not "super saints", just weak vessels God chooses to use.

Look for His Mercies

"Because of the Lord's great love we are not consumed, for His compassions never fail. They are new every morning; great is your faithfulness." Lamentations 3:22-23

Never have I experienced God's mercies as I did when Day lay dying in a nursing home. His night nurse was a very special young man. We had a wonderful hospice team those last two weeks of his life as well.

We had been keeping a bedside vigil, but he had not changed, so we all went home to rest. At 1:00am we were called back to the nursing home. At 10:00am, every member of our hospice team arrived to share Dan's last moments. They were there to guide us through each step after he died, and to hug us in our grief.

Dan died on December 29. My brother was on Christmas break from the Bible college where he teaches, and was able to come and do the memorial service.

Dan had a short nursing home stay; only five weeks. I had family living with me. I had an inheritance with which I was able to pay the nursing home care. God showered on us one mercy after another.

Action Step: Look for God's mercies. They are new every morning and there is a special mercy for each hour.

Isolation

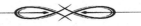

"While he himself went a day's journey into the desert. He came to a broom tree, sat down under it and prayed that he might die. 'I have had enough, Lord,' he said. 'Take my life. I am no better than my ancestors.'" 1 Kings 19:4

Alzheimer's tends to isolate us as we must stay home to care for our loved one. We can't take long trips anymore. We took our last long trip the year before Dan died. I never closed my daycare and Dan loved our little ones. We continued to go to church and growth group, as well as do our prayer group at the prison. We did all of this until six weeks before Dan died.

What I visualized never happened: that I would have to close the daycare and be confined to my home caring for Dan. But situations like that do happen.

There are volunteer organizations out there that will

send someone to be with your loved one and give you a break. Use them.

Dan even went shopping with me the last Saturday, but he ran the grocery cart into a shelf and broke some glassware. That was the end of that. He would be hospitalized that Sunday and later moved to the nursing home. Some decisions just make themselves.

Action Step: If you become isolated, do what you need to do to have a break away from the care of your loved one.

Wait on the Lord

"But they that wait upon the Lord shall renew their strength; they shall mount up on wings as eagles, they shall run and not be weary, and they shall walk and not grow faint." Isaiah 40:31

What does it mean to wait upon the Lord? I believe it means spending time with Him saturating your soul with the word, meditating on the verses, praying, and listening. You can come away from a quiet time like that renewed and ready for whatever your day brings.

You can literally get exhausted as a caregiver. Toward the last weeks I cared for Dan, he was getting me up four and five times a night. The interrupted sleep took its toll on me. Even going to the nursing home every night to feed him and spend time with him wore me out.

There is no substitute for time alone with God. You need

the renewing of your strength, so you can meet the demands of your responsibilities.

A verse in a song, a phrase, a quote, can be food for your soul. You need that time in God's throne room.

Things can be very unpredictable with an Alzheimer's patient. Don't be surprised by anything. And maybe even find humor in it.

Action Step: Spend time with God before your day begins. You will gain much needed strength for the demands of your day.

Touch is so Important

❦

"Jesus reached out His hand and touched the man. 'I am willing,' he said. 'Be clean!' Immediately he was cured of his leprosy." Matthew 8:3

Touch is so important with an Alzheimer's patient. When words can't reach them anymore, touch can. Take their hand. Give a hug. Be aware of your tone of voice.

Have you noticed how many times Jesus touched someone in the gospels? He even touched a leper.

Once in awhile, my mom would have a crying spell while I was caring for her. She couldn't tell me what was wrong, and I couldn't figure it out. I would just sit beside her on the bed and put my arms around her until she quieted.

Nathan sat beside his father's bed, holding his hand as he was taking his last breaths.

Jesus raised Jarius' daughter to life after touching her hand. He made clay and touched a blind man's eyes. He washed and his sight was returned to him.

Those hugs by the hospice team immediately after Dan died meant so much. I love hugs. Dan and I used to have a hug every morning to start our day. Remember to touch. It is more important than you realize.

Action Step: Touch often. It means much more than your words. With words there is a chance they may not reach your loved one, but touch, breaks all barriers.

Be Kind

"Be kind and compassionate to one another, forgiving each other, just as Christ forgave you." Ephesians 4:32

As you care for your loved one, God begins to bring forth the fruit of His spirit in your life in a new way. I knew when Dan got Alzheimer's He was working on gentleness in my life. I'm not a very gentle person, but I knew I would become gentler through the process of caring for my husband. Kindness and compassion are not far behind.

God is known for His loving-kindness. That word is not used for anyone else. When Paul prayed for the Ephesians, he prayed that they would come to know God's love in such a way that they would be filled with the fullness of God. If God is filled with loving-kindness, and we are filled with the fullness of God, then we can show His loving-kindness to those we care for. Awesome thought.

I prayed while I was in Israel that God would so fill me with His love that it would spill out to all around me, and He did just that.

You are commanded to be kind, and kindness is one of the fruits of the spirit within you.

Action Step: As a caregiver, be kind and compassionate to your loved one. It will pay great dividends.

Praises at Midnight

"After they had been severely flogged, they were thrown in jail and the jailor was commanded to guard them carefully. About midnight, Paul and Silas were praying and singing hymns to God, and the other prisoners were listening to them."
Acts 16: 23,25

Paul and Silas were in the city of Phillipi. Paul had cast out a demon from a young woman, and her irate owners dragged Paul and Silas before the authorities. They were severely beaten, put in prison, and their feet put into stocks. With bleeding and bruised backs, feet locked up, fighting sleeplessness, Paul and Silas held a midnight prayer meeting and began to sing praises to God. Then, suddenly, there was an earthquake and everyone's chains were loosed, and the prison doors flew open. Paul called out to the jailor that no one had escaped. That night, the jailor and his entire family came to know the Lord.

Dan lay dying in a nursing home. Nathan, John, and I kept vigil by his bedside. On Tuesday, Nathan borrowed a guitar and we all sang praises around his bed, all day long. Two days later, I would say goodbye to Dan on earth. But, that special day of praise would stick in my memory.

Action Step: Learn to praise God in the midnights of life, however, whenever they come, and no matter how painful they may be.

When I am Weak

"But he said to me, 'My grace is sufficient for you, for my power is made perfect in weakness. Therefore, I will boast all the more gladly about my weaknesses, so that Christ's power may rest on me." 2 Corinthians 12:9

When you are at your weakest, God's power is most manifest. God delights in using weak people. Now it may take a great deal of faith and grace to actually boast in your weakness as Paul did.

When my brother was so ill, I prayed these verses for him. He confessed, "I don't think I am to the point of boasting about my weaknesses yet."

I'm 71, and full of arthritis, and don't have much energy. When God called me to go to Israel as a volunteer, I said, "You are sending a very weak vessel, but I will go." God, amazingly, gave me the strength I needed.

Dear caregiver, your loved ones' weakness may become your strength. God is building His character in you through caring for your loved one. The fruits of love, joy, patience, kindness, and gentleness increasingly grow in your garden. You are changed through another's weakness.

Action Step: Realize your loved one's weakness becomes your strength as God forms His character in you, through your caregiving.

That Black Hole

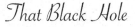

*"I called your name, O Lord, from the depths of the pit. You
heard my plea; Do not close your ears to my cry for relief.
You came near when I called you and you said, 'Do not fear.'"*
Lamentations 3:55-57

Jeremiah had many enemies. They were tired of hearing
of the coming judgment. So they did a cruel thing: they
put Jeremiah in an empty cistern, put the lid on it, and left
him there. Jeremiah sank down in the mire and mud in
the darkness. He cried out to God and God met him there
in the darkness, saying: "Fear not. I am with you." But
someone saw what they did to Jeremiah and rescued him.

When one has Alzheimer's or memory loss, there are
times of darkness. You may feel like you are sinking into
a black hole. You may not even be able to find the words
to pray and cry out to God. He hears the words you can't

utter. He feels your heart need, and He comes with a gentle whisper, telling us: "Fear not. I am with you. Take my hand in the darkness, and feel my presence." And, in His kindness, He will draw you out of the pit, and set your feet on solid ground once more.

Action Step: When the darkness comes, cry out to God. He will hear your cry and come to you, and you will hear His gentle whisper: "Fear not. I am with you."

Contentment

───────✦✦───────

*"I know what it is to be in need, and I know what it is to have
plenty. I have learned the secret to being content in any and
every situation, whether well-fed or hungry, whether living in
plenty or in want." Philippians 4:12*

Contentment is a learned response, and it does not

come easily. Can you be content in the midst of Alzhei-

mer's? Can you be content to be the caregiver? Situations

are going to rise that are going to be difficult. Can both of

you be content in them? Can you give thanks in the midst

of the trial?

Your faith will be tested in many ways. Will you cling to

God and stand firm? Will you run to Him for refuge? For

comfort?

Hand your frustration to God. Alzheimer's is a disease

of losses, and I grieved each one. When they removed

Dan from his position as prison chaplain, and took his classes away. When he could no longer take inmates to the bus. When he could no longer drive.

I think to really be content, we have to be thankful in everything. God didn't say living the Christian life would be easy, but it would be worth it.

Action Step: Practice and learn contentment in each and every circumstance, giving thanks always.

Comfort

> *"Praise be to the God and Father of our Lord Jesus Christ,*
> *the Father of compassion and the God of all comfort, who*
> *comforts us in all our troubles, so that we can comfort those in*
> *any trouble, with the comfort we ourselves have received from*
> *God." 2 Corinthians 1:3-4*

As I have shared my journey through Dan's Alzheimer's with you, I hope I have shared how God comforted me.

Do you realize the entire Trinity comforts us, both caregiver and patient? Here, the Father is called the God of all comfort. When Jesus left earth, He sent the Holy Spirit, and called Him the comforter. Jesus is our great high priest, and also comforts us.

Have you taken a young child in your arms and comforted them when they hurt themselves? I do it often in my daycare. God does the same for us when we are hurting. He may bring a verse of scripture to our mind with just the right words we need to hear, or the words of a hymn, or the counsel of a friend. Perhaps someone will pray with us over the phone, and our spirits are lifted.

One totally stressed out day, I had three different people pray with me over the phone, and I was comforted.

Action Step: Just crawl up in the lap of God, and pour out your heart and be comforted.

Use Music

⟫⟨⟩⟫

"He put a new song in my mouth, a hymn of praise to my
God. Many will see and fear, and put their trust in the Lord."
Psalm 40:3

Music was such a huge part of my mother's life. She had

graduated from college with a degree in music, taught

music, and directed a church choir for many years. When

she could no longer speak an intelligent word, she could

still sing the old hymns.

A friend shared how her father, disabled by several

strokes, could still sing the songs he loved, though he

couldn't actually talk. They even gave him an ipod so he

could have music during his wheelchair outings.

So use music, especially the old hymns or even newer

worship choruses. There is much comfort in music, and

scriptural truth that ministers to our hearts.

God has often brought the words of an old hymn to my mind when He wanted to remind me of a truth that I needed at that moment.

When I write, I put a CD of easy-listening classical music in. When I was so depressed, I listened to the same tape of Christian music ever morning and was encouraged.

Action Step: Ask God to put a new song in your heart, even praise unto your God. Put on a CD and fill your heart and home with praise music.

God is a Finisher

———✦———

*"In all my prayers for all of you, I always pray with joy…
being confident of this: that He who began a good work in you
will carry it on to completion until the day of Christ Jesus."*
Philippians 1:4-6

What a comfort in this life to know God is going to
complete His work in our hearts and lives. That nothing
can hinder that work from being finished and perfected.
Not memory loss, not even physical weakness that sets us
aside for a season. That just being God's child and resting
in His loving arms is enough. That through my very weakness, God's purposes for me are being accomplished. That
through my weakness, others learn to be true servants
to God as they care for me. God may be accomplishing
more through my days of being cared for than when I was
actively serving Him.

I still took Dan to the prison when he could no longer talk and make sense. His presence and his smile were enough, and he could still shake hands with the men he loved. Just his presence ministered to the men. Even in the nursing home, his sweet spirit ministered to those who cared for him.

Action Step: God is still fulfilling His purposes for you, even through your weaknesses. Just rest in His loving arms.

I Will Strengthen You

❦

"So do not fear, for I am with you; do not be dismayed, for I am your God. I will strengthen you and help you; I will uphold you with my righteous right hand." Isaiah 41:10

Whether you are the caregiver, or the loved one being cared for, you need strength and the presence of God to get through the days. Let's look at Isaiah 41:10, phrase by phrase.

"Fear not, for I am with you." Let me quiet the dread within your heart by my loving presence."

"Be not dismayed; for I am your God." Don't lose courage in the face of these alarming prospects, for I am your personal God. I care about you, and I'm in control of every detail of your lives.

"I will strengthen you." I'll make you strong to bear the

days ahead. I will give you courage for when you are weak, and I'll be your strength.

"I will uphold you with my righteous right hand." I will raise you up when you are bowed down with struggle. I will sustain and keep you, encouraging you with my victorious right hand. My purpose is to make you triumph over your difficulties, and I have the power to make that happen. Place your hand in mine, and together we will tread each step into the future.

Action Step: Start each day seeking God's help and strength. The whole day will go better if you do.

God's Invitation

"Come to me, all you who are weary and heavy-laden, and I will give you rest. Take my yoke upon you, and learn from me. For I am gentle and humble in heart, and you will find rest for your souls. For my yoke is easy and my burden is light."
Matthew 11:28-30

Are you just plain worn out with your caregiving? Weary to the bone? Too tired to go on? Without the spiritual resources that have been outlined here?

Listen carefully to Jesus' invitation. It is for you personally. Come to Him. Give your life to Him and let Him take over the controls. He will give you that rest for your soul that you need.

Step into God's forever family by believing Jesus died for your sins on the cross. That He bore your death penalty and in return gives you eternal life.

Exchange your heavy yoke for His easy one, your heavy burden for His light one.

Place your hand in His and together, tread into the future. He will fill you with His faith, love, joy, and peace. His Holy Spirit comes to dwell within you and you now have all the spiritual resources you need.

Action Step: Come to Jesus now. Find your rest in Him. Place your feet on the path to heaven.

Devotions

For the Patient

The Comforter

"But I tell you the truth, it is for your good that I am going away. Unless I go away, the Counselor will not come to you; but if I go, I will send him to you." John 16:7

If you are the patient struggling with Alzheimer's, you need to remember that God's Holy Spirit dwells within you. He is called the comforter, the One who comes alongside to help. He is in total control of your subconscious mind, and can bring to the surface just the thoughts and words needed for whatever moment lies before you.

I read a book written by a pastor with Alzheimer's in which the pastor described how the Holy Spirit broke through the fog with incredible comfort and love.

Just rest yourself in the arms of God, dear one. He is still there and can break through when you least expect it. He made your mind and He is still in control, even when you feel you are losing it. Trust yourself to God and let Him fill in the blanks.

One instance, when I was caring for my mom, I found her struggling to put in her partial plate. When she finally accomplished it, she exclaimed: "Praise the Lord!" What a surprise from a mother who couldn't make sense when she spoke anymore.

Insight: The God who made your mind gave you His Holy Spirit who will meet your needs moment by moment.

When I am Gray-Headed

"Even to your old age, I am He; and even to gray hairs I will carry you. I have made, and I will bear, and I will carry, and I will deliver you." Isaiah 46: 4

I want you to know, God is never going to forsake you. Even in the gray-headed years. God will be there for you. When you are weak, when your mind fails you, God will carry you through and bring you safely home to glory. There you will be perfect, with a mind that will work even better than it did here on earth.

David cried out: "Don't take me away until I've declared your mighty works to the generation to come! Until I've shared your faithfulness to my children and grandchildren." (Psalm 71:18)

When you can no longer walk, when you can no longer

speak, God will still minister through you to those who care for you.

Dan was so easy to care for that the nurses loved caring for him. He was still fulfilling God's plan for his life, even in his weakness.

God carried him, and He carried us, through those days. It was really difficult to see him there, in that nursing home, but I grew to appreciate those who cared for him.

Insight: Even in your gray-headed years, God will never forsake you. He will carry you until you are safely home.

Our Great High Priest

"*For we do not have a high priest who is unable to sympathize with our weaknesses, but we have one who has been tempted in every way, just as we are, yet was without sin.*"
Hebrews 4:15

There is nothing we can go through on this earth that Jesus has not been through before us. And, because He has, He can feel our pain with us. He knew frustration, anger, misunderstanding, discouragement, depression. He also walked through the valley of death. He may not have lost His mind, but they accused Him of it, saying: "Are you mad, calling yourself the Son of God?"

What touches you, touches Him, and He knows how to pray for you, and comfort you. People around you may not understand, but Jesus has perfect understanding. He knows just what word to whisper in your ear.

Run to the throne of grace and receive the mercy and grace for your time of need. Grace received is simply the ability to do it God's way; forgiving those who have hurt you and simply don't understand how difficult your path is.

God gives grace for the trials, unfailing sympathy, undying love. Rest in Him.

Insight: Put your hand in Jesus' hand, and walk this path through Alzheimer's together. He will never fail you.

Kept by His Power

"To Him who is able to keep you from falling, and who presents you before His glorious presence without fault and with great joy..." Jude 24

God is never going to let you down or fail you. He has a goal for your life, and He will see it through to completion.

There is a great presentation ceremony for you one day in heaven. No matter how weak you become, God Himself will keep you from falling, and present you spotless before the throne with great joy.

You are God's pride and joy, and He will not let anything happen to spoil that presentation.

He will surround you with loving caregivers, until their work is done and you graduate to glory. His mercies will be new every day, and His compassions fail not. You will still be serving Him in your weakness as you allow others to care for you. For God is working in their lives through your weakness.

I was brokenhearted when I couldn't care for Dan anymore. I stood by his bed and said with tears in my eyes: "I can't care for you anymore." But God put many caring people in my place.

Insight: All you have to do is be yourself and let God care for you through your caregivers. Your weakness makes them better servants.

Underneath are the Everlasting Arms

"The eternal God is your refuge, and underneath are the everlasting arms. He will drive out your enemy before you saying, 'Destroy him!'" Deuteronomy 35:27

Remember this, dear one, you can never fall out of God's arms. Those everlasting arms are always under you, lovingly carrying you.

Remember the poem "Footprints"? When there were two sets of footprints, that is when, hand in hand, you were walking with Jesus. When there was only one set of footprints, you thought He had deserted you. But He answered: "That was when I carried you."

When we grow old and weak and our mind goes, God is still there. He has not deserted us. He cannot, for His eternal presence is with us, inside the person of the Holy Spirit.

So rest in Him. Let go, and let God. The eternal God is thy refuge. Run to Him and be safe. Rest in those loving arms. Put your head on His breast and feel the beating of His heart for you.

Can you take pleasure in your weakness knowing Christ's power rests on you? You are still fulfilling God's plan for you, even though someone else must care for you. God is building in your caregiver, through you, His character.

Insight: Rejoice in your infirmities, for God's strength shows up best in your weakness.

This Momentary Trouble

"For our light and momentary troubles are achieving for us eternal glory that far outweighs them all. So we fix our eyes not on what is seen, but on what is unseen. For what is seen is temporal, but what is unseen is eternal." 2 Corinthians 4:17-18

Paul suffered so much for the sake of the gospel. How did he endure so much suffering? Because he had divine connection and was renewed inwardly day by day. He calls these outward trials "light and momentary troubles." He fixed his eyes on the eternal glory those very troubles would bring one day, knowing outward things would soon pass away.

We must do the same. The secret is keeping our eyes on Jesus, not our circumstances, or what is happening to our body. It is praying from God to our circumstances, not from our circumstances to God. There is a huge difference.

I must keep reminding myself: "God you are the blessed controller of all things, even though I see my son making foolish decisions. You love him just as much as you love me, and you are at work in his life."

So, no matter what is happening outwardly, keep your eyes heavenward.

Insight: Focus on the eternal, not the temporal. On eternal glory, not temporary loss.

Safe in His Love

"For I am convinced, that neither death nor life, neither angels, nor demons, neither the present nor the future, nor any powers, neither height nor depth, nor anything else in all creation, will be able to separate us from the love of God that is in Christ Jesus our Lord." Romans 8:38-39

Dear one, no matter what happens, you are safe in God's great love. Absolutely nothing can separate you from that love. Even if you lose your mind completely, and you don't know anyone, God still knows you and loves you with an everlasting love. There is nothing that can happen today or tomorrow that can separate you from that love.

You are God's precious child and He cares for you as only God can. You are completely protected and secure in His love.

My prayer for you is that God would so wrap you in His loving-kindness and mercy that you will be free of fear; that He would be such a refuge for you, that you can rest in the unknown without anxiety. That your weakness will become your caregiver's strength. That God will be glorified in your life, all the way through your battle with Alzheimer's.

Insight: Rest in the security and certainty of God's love for you.

The More Feeble are Necessary

"On the contrary, those parts of the body that seem to be weaker are indispensable, and the parts that we think are less honorable, we treat with special honor..."
1 Corinthians 12:22-23

Did you know that in your weakness you are absolutely necessary to the body of Christ? Once you actively served Christ, but now you feel useless. You are still fulfilling your part in the body of Christ, even as you are cared for.

You are teaching others how to be true servants to Christ by your weaknesses. We learn to show Christ's love in new ways, and those who observe our love for you are drawn to Christ. We become more compassionate, kind, gentle, patient, and long-suffering. We learn to put up with things in new ways. We are stretched, and we grow through caring for you.

I watched a man whose wife was in a wheel chair. He faithfully got her ready and brought her to church every Sunday. As his loving care for her is observed, we, as care-givers, are touched. I greeted another elderly woman in her wheel chair each Sunday, and love and bless her. She always placed her hand in mine, and smiled at me. Yes, the more feeble are necessary to the body of Christ. They have so much to teach us as we care for them.

Insight: They also serve who only stand and wait. You "be" and we will serve and care for you.

CPSIA information can be obtained
at www.ICGtesting.com
Printed in the USA
LVOW13s1048020317
525929LV00015B/415/P